I0767416

CHRISTOPHER MORRIS

Chronic Pain Relief: Strategies for Wellness and Healing

Chronic pain

First published by Christopher Morris 2024

Copyright © 2024 by christopher morris

All rights reserved. No part of this publication may be reproduced, stored or transmitted in any form or by any means, electronic, mechanical, photocopying, recording, scanning, or otherwise without written permission from the publisher. It is illegal to copy this book, post it to a website, or distribute it by any other means without permission.

christopher morris asserts the moral right to be identified as the author of this work.

christopher morris has no responsibility for the persistence or accuracy of URLs for external or third-party Internet Websites referred to in this publication and does not guarantee that any content on such Websites is, or will remain, accurate or appropriate.

First edition

This book was professionally typeset on Reedsy.
Find out more at reedsy.com

Contents

1 Chapter 1: Introduction 1

2 Chapter 2: Understanding Chronic Pain 4

3 Chapter 3: Traditional Treatments for Chronic Pain 7

4 Chapter 4: Nutrition and Chronic Pain 10

5 Chapter 5: Exercise and Chronic Pain 14

6 Chapter 6: Mind-Body Connection 18

7 Chapter 7: Creating a Holistic Pain Management Plan 21

8 Chapter 8: Alternative Therapies for Chronic Pain 24

9 Chapter 9: Sleep and Chronic Pain 27

10 Chapter 10: Technology and Chronic Pain Management 31

11 Chapter 11: Herbal Remedies and Supplements for Pain Relief 35

12 Chapter 12: Support Systems for Coping with Chronic Pain 39

13 Chapter 13: Lifestyle Modifications for Pain Management 42

14 Chapter 14: Spirituality and Chronic Pain 46

15 Chapter 15: Advocacy and Empowerment in Pain Management 49

16 Chapter 16: Long-Term Strategies for Maintaining Pain Relief 53

17 Chapter 17: Coping Techniques for Flare-Ups and Setbacks   57

18 Chapter 18: Exploring Energy Healing Modalities for Pain...   60

19 Chapter 19: Integrative Approaches to Pain Management ...   63

20 Chapter 20: The Role of Sleep Hygiene in Chronic Pain...   66

21 Chapter 21: Utilizing Cognitive-Behavioral Therapy for Pain...   70

22 Chapter 22: Art Therapy and Creative Expression in Pain...   73

23 Chapter 23: Financial Wellness and Chronic Pain: Navigating...   76

24 Chapter 24: Animal-Assisted Therapy for Chronic Pain...   80

25 Chapter 25: The Science of Pain: Understanding Neurological...   83

26 Chapter:26 References   87

27 Chapter:27 Conclusion   91

1

Chapter 1: Introduction

Chronic pain is a complex and pervasive issue that affects millions of individuals worldwide. Unlike acute pain, which typically resolves with time and treatment, chronic pain persists for an extended period – often lasting for months or even years. It can have a significant impact on a person's physical, mental, and emotional well-being, leading to decreased quality of life, reduced productivity, and increased healthcare costs.

Overview of Chronic Pain

Chronic pain can manifest in a variety of ways, including sharp or stabbing pain, dull aches, burning sensations, or throbbing discomfort. It can affect any part of the body, from the head to the toes, and may be caused by a wide range of underlying conditions such as arthritis, fibromyalgia, nerve damage, or injury. The intensity and frequency of chronic pain can vary from person to person, making it a highly individualized experience.

One of the key challenges in managing chronic pain is the

subjective nature of the condition. Unlike acute pain, which is typically a symptom of an injury or illness, chronic pain can persist long after the initial cause has been addressed. This can make it difficult to diagnose and treat effectively, leading to frustration for both patients and healthcare providers.

Importance of Holistic Approaches for Pain Management

Given the complexity of chronic pain, a holistic approach to pain management is essential for providing effective and comprehensive care to individuals suffering from this condition. Holistic therapies focus on addressing the physical, emotional, and psychological aspects of pain, rather than just treating the symptoms. By taking a holistic approach, healthcare providers can help patients manage their pain more effectively and improve their overall quality of life.

One of the key benefits of holistic pain management is its focus on treating the whole person, rather than just the pain itself. This can involve a combination of conventional medical treatments, such as medications or physical therapy, along with complementary therapies, such as acupuncture, massage, or mindfulness techniques. By addressing the physical, emotional, and psychological aspects of pain, holistic approaches can help patients achieve greater pain relief and improve their overall well-being.

In addition to providing more comprehensive care, holistic approaches to pain management can also help reduce the risk of dependence on pain medications and minimize the potential for adverse side effects. By combining a variety of therapies and techniques, healthcare providers can help patients find relief from their pain without relying solely on pharmaceutical interventions. This can be particularly important for individuals who are at risk for addiction or other complications associated with long-term medication use.

Furthermore, holistic approaches to pain management can empower patients to take an active role in their care. By incorporating self-care strategies, such as exercise, nutrition, stress management, and mind-body techniques, patients can learn how to better manage their pain on a day-to-day basis. This can lead to improved pain control, reduced reliance on healthcare providers, and a greater sense of empowerment and control over their health.

In conclusion, chronic pain is a complex and challenging condition that requires a multifaceted approach to management. By incorporating holistic therapies and techniques into pain management plans, healthcare providers can help patients achieve greater pain relief, improve their overall quality of life, and reduce the risk of dependence on medications. Through a combination of conventional and complementary therapies, patients can find relief from their pain and regain control over their health and well-being.

2

Chapter 2: Understanding Chronic Pain

Chronic pain is a complex and pervasive condition that affects millions of individuals worldwide. Defined as pain that persists for an extended period, typically lasting for at least three to six months, chronic pain can have a profound impact on an individual's quality of life. Unlike acute pain, which serves as a warning signal to the body that something is wrong, chronic pain persists long after the initial injury or illness has healed. This can lead to a cycle of pain and disability that can be challenging to break.

Common chronic pain conditions include arthritis, fibromyalgia, and back pain. Arthritis is a condition that causes inflammation in the joints, leading to pain, stiffness, and swelling. It can affect any joint in the body but is most found in the hands, knees, hips, and spine. Fibromyalgia is a chronic condition characterized by widespread musculoskeletal pain, fatigue, and tender points throughout the body. Back pain is a common issue that can be caused by a variety of factors, including muscle strain, injury, or underlying medical conditions.

The impact of chronic pain on physical and mental health can be significant. In addition to the constant presence of pain, individuals with chronic pain may experience fatigue, sleep disturbances, and difficulty performing daily activities. Chronic pain can also lead to feelings of anxiety, depression, and isolation. The burden of chronic pain can be overwhelming, affecting an individual's ability to work, engage in social activities, and maintain relationships. This can lead to a decreased quality of life and a sense of hopelessness.

Physical health can also be affected by chronic pain. Individuals with chronic pain may be less likely to engage in physical activity, leading to a decline in physical fitness and an increased risk of developing other health conditions. Furthermore, chronic pain can impact the immune system, making individuals more susceptible to infections and other illnesses. Chronic pain can also lead to changes in brain chemistry, increasing the risk of developing conditions such as depression and anxiety.

Understanding chronic pain is essential to effectively manage and treat this complex condition. While there is no single cause of chronic pain, it is believed to be influenced by a combination of factors, including genetics, lifestyle, and environmental factors. Chronic pain is a multifaceted experience that involves physical, emotional, and psychological components. Individuals with chronic pain need to seek out comprehensive care that addresses all aspects of their condition.

Treatment options for chronic pain vary depending on the under-lying cause and severity of the pain. Common treatments may include medications, physical therapy, psychological counseling, and alternative therapies such as acupuncture or massage. Individuals with chronic pain need to work closely with their healthcare providers to develop a comprehensive treatment plan that addresses their unique needs and goals.

In conclusion, chronic pain is a complex and challenging condition that can have a significant impact on an individual's physical and mental health. Understanding the nature of chronic pain, common chronic pain conditions, and the impact of chronic pain on physical and mental health is essential to effectively manage and treat this condition. By working closely with healthcare providers and exploring a variety of treatment options, individuals with chronic pain can improve their quality of life and find relief from their symptoms.

3

Chapter 3: Traditional Treatments for Chronic Pain

Chronic pain is a debilitating condition that affects millions of people worldwide. Traditional treatments for chronic pain encompass a variety of options, including medication, physical therapy, and surgery. Each of these treatment modalities has its own set of benefits and limitations, which patients and healthcare providers must carefully consider when devising a comprehensive pain management plan.

Overview of Traditional Pain Management Options

Medication is one of the most common forms of treatment for chronic pain. Nonsteroidal anti-inflammatory drugs (NSAIDs), such as ibuprofen, can help reduce inflammation and alleviate pain. Opioids, like oxycodone and morphine, are often pre-scribed for severe pain but come with the risk of addiction and other serious side effects. Antidepressants and anticonvulsants can also be used to manage certain types of chronic pain.

Physical therapy is another important component of traditional pain management. Physical therapists can design individualized exercise programs to help improve strength, flexibility, and range of motion. They may also use techniques such as massage, heat therapy, and electrical stimulation to alleviate pain and promote healing.

In some cases, surgery may be necessary to address the underlying cause of chronic pain. Procedures such as joint replacement, spinal fusion, and nerve decompression can provide long-lasting relief for certain conditions. However, surgery is not without risks, and patients must carefully weigh the potential benefits against the potential complications.

Benefits and Limitations of Traditional Treatments

Medication can be an effective way to manage chronic pain, particularly in the short term. NSAIDs and opioids can provide immediate relief from pain, allowing patients to resume their daily activities. However, long-term use of opioids can lead to tolerance, dependence, and addiction, while NSAIDs can cause gastrointestinal ulcers and kidney damage.

Physical therapy offers a non-invasive approach to pain management that focuses on improving function and quality of life. By targeting specific muscle groups and joints, physical therapists can help patients reduce pain and improve their overall physical health. However, physical therapy can be time-consuming and may not provide immediate relief for all patients.

Surgery is often reserved for cases of chronic pain that do

not respond to other treatments. While surgery can be highly effective at addressing the underlying cause of pain, it is also associated with several risks, including infection, nerve damage, and prolonged recovery times. Additionally, surgery may not always eliminate pain and can sometimes lead to new or worsened pain.

In conclusion, traditional treatments for chronic pain offer a range of options for patients seeking relief from their symptoms. Medication, physical therapy, and surgery each have their own set of benefits and limitations, and patients must work closely with their healthcare providers to determine the best course of treatment for their individual needs. By carefully weighing the risks and benefits of each treatment modality, patients can make informed decisions about their pain management plan and work towards improving their quality of life.

4

Chapter 4: Nutrition and Chronic Pain

Nutrition plays a crucial role in managing chronic pain. While medication and therapy are commonly used to alleviate pain, the foods we consume can also have a significant impact on our pain levels. In this chapter, we will explore the role of diet in managing chronic pain, including foods to avoid and foods to include for pain relief, as well as the use of nutritional supplements for pain management.

The Role of Diet in Managing Chronic Pain

The foods we eat can either exacerbate or alleviate chronic pain. Processed foods high in sugar, sodium, and unhealthy fats can increase inflammation in the body, leading to worsened pain symptoms. On the other hand, whole foods rich in antioxidants, vitamins, and minerals can help reduce inflammation and provide relief from pain.

Incorporating a balanced diet rich in fruits, vegetables, whole grains, lean proteins, and healthy fats can help manage chronic pain. These foods provide essential nutrients that support overall health and can help reduce inflammation, which is often a key driver of chronic pain conditions.

Foods to Avoid and Foods to Include for Pain Relief

When it comes to managing chronic pain through diet, there are certain foods to avoid and others to include for pain relief. Foods to avoid include processed foods, sugary beverages, fried foods, and foods high in trans fats. These foods can increase inflammation in the body and worsen pain symptoms.

On the other hand, foods to include for pain relief include:

Fatty fish: Rich in omega-3 fatty acids, fatty fish like salmon, mackerel, and sardines have anti-inflammatory properties that can help reduce pain.

Berries: Berries like blueberries, strawberries, and blackberries are packed with antioxidants that can help reduce inflammation and provide relief from pain.

Leafy greens: Leafy greens like spinach, kale, and Swiss chard are rich in vitamins and minerals that support overall health and can help reduce inflammation.

Nuts and seeds: Nuts and seeds like almonds, walnuts, and chia seeds are high in healthy fats and antioxidants that can help alleviate pain.

Turmeric: Turmeric contains curcumin, a compound with powerful anti-inflammatory properties that can help reduce pain and inflammation.

Incorporating these foods into your diet can help manage chronic pain and improve overall health.

Nutritional Supplements for Pain Management

In addition to incorporating pain-relieving foods into your diet, nutritional supplements can also be beneficial for managing chronic pain. Some of the most used supplements for pain management include:

Omega-3 fatty acids: Fish oil supplements are a popular choice for reducing inflammation and alleviating pain.

Vitamin D: Low levels of vitamin D have been linked to increased pain sensitivity, so supplementing with vitamin D can help manage pain symptoms.

Magnesium: Magnesium plays a key role in muscle relaxation and can help alleviate muscle pain and stiffness.

Curcumin: Curcumin supplements, derived from turmeric, can help reduce inflammation and provide relief from pain.

Glucosamine and chondroitin: These supplements are commonly used to support joint health and reduce pain associated with conditions like osteoarthritis.

Before starting any nutritional supplements for pain management, it is important to consult with a healthcare provider to ensure they are safe and appropriate for your individual needs.

In conclusion, nutrition plays a crucial role in managing chronic pain. By incorporating a balanced diet rich in whole foods and pain-relieving nutrients, avoiding inflammatory foods, and considering the use of nutritional supplements, you can help alleviate pain symptoms and improve overall health. By taking a holistic approach to pain management that includes both traditional treatments and dietary changes, you can better manage chronic pain and live a more fulfilling life.

5

Chapter 5: Exercise and Chronic Pain

Exercise is often considered one of the best natural remedies for chronic pain relief. While it may seem counterintuitive to move when experiencing pain, research has shown that engaging in regular physical activity can help alleviate symptoms and improve overall quality of life for individuals suffering from chronic pain conditions.

Benefits of exercise for chronic pain relief

There is a multitude of benefits associated with incorporating exercise into a treatment plan for chronic pain. Some of these benefits include:

Increased endorphin production: Exercise has been shown to stimulate the production of endorphins, which are the body's natural painkillers. These endorphins can help reduce the perception of pain and improve mood.

Improved muscle strength and flexibility: Chronic pain conditions often lead to muscle weakness and stiffness. Regular exercise can help strengthen muscles, improve flexibility, and reduce the risk of further injury.

Enhanced circulation: Exercise can help improve blood flow to the muscles and joints, which can aid in reducing inflammation and promoting healing.

Weight management: Maintaining a healthy weight is crucial for managing chronic pain conditions such as osteoarthritis and back pain. Regular exercise can help individuals achieve and maintain a healthy weight, which can in turn reduce the strain on their joints and muscles.

Better sleep quality: Chronic pain is often associated with sleep disturbances. Engaging in regular physical activity can help regulate sleep patterns and improve overall sleep quality.

Types of exercises recommended for different chronic pain conditions.

The type of exercise recommended for chronic pain relief will vary depending on the individual's specific condition and needs. Some common types of exercises that are often recommended for different chronic pain conditions include:

Low-impact aerobic exercises: Activities such as walking, swimming, and cycling are excellent options for individuals with chronic pain conditions such as osteoarthritis and fibromyalgia. These exercises help improve cardiovascular health and promote overall well-being without putting excessive strain on the joints.

Strength training: Building muscle strength is crucial for individuals with chronic pain conditions that affect the muscles and joints. Incorporating exercises such as weightlifting, resistance band workouts, and bodyweight exercises can help improve muscle tone and reduce pain.

Stretching exercises: Stretching exercises such as yoga and Pilates can help improve flexibility, reduce muscle stiffness, and alleviate pain associated with conditions such as back pain and arthritis.

Mind-body exercises: Activities such as tai chi and qigong combine physical movement with mindfulness and relaxation techniques. These practices can help reduce stress, improve mental clarity, and promote healing for individuals with chronic pain conditions.

Tips for incorporating physical activity into daily routine.

Incorporating exercise into a daily routine can be challenging, especially for individuals dealing with chronic pain. However, with some careful planning and dedication, it is possible to make physical activity a regular part of one's lifestyle. Some tips for incorporating exercise into a daily routine include:

Start slow: Begin with gentle exercises and gradually increase intensity and duration as your fitness level improves. Listen to your body and avoid pushing yourself too hard.

Set realistic goals: Establish achievable goals for your exercise routine and track your progress. Celebrate small victories along the way to stay motivated.

Find activities you enjoy: Choose exercises that you find enjoyable and engaging. Whether it's dancing, gardening, or hiking, find activities that bring you joy and make you want to move.

Schedule workouts: Set aside dedicated time for exercise in

your daily schedule. Treat it like any other appointment and prioritize your physical health.

Seek professional guidance: Consider working with a physical therapist or personal trainer who can tailor an exercise program to meet your specific needs and goals.

In conclusion, exercise is a powerful tool for managing chronic pain and improving overall well-being. By incorporating regular physical activity into your daily routine and choosing exercises that are safe and effective for your specific condition, you can experience significant relief from pain and enjoy a better quality of life. Remember to listen to your body, set realistic goals, and seek professional guidance when needed to make the most of your exercise regimen.

6

Chapter 6: Mind-Body Connection

The mind-body connection is a powerful and intricate relationship that plays a crucial role in our overall well-being. In the context of chronic pain, this connection becomes especially important as mental health can greatly impact the experience of pain. Understanding the link between mental health and chronic pain, as well as learning techniques for managing stress and anxiety related to pain, can greatly improve an individual's quality of life.

The Link Between Mental Health and Chronic Pain

Chronic pain is not just a physical sensation; it also has a significant impact on one's mental health. Studies have shown that individuals experiencing chronic pain are more likely to also suffer from depression, anxiety, and other psychological disorders. The constant presence of pain can lead to feelings of helplessness, frustration, and isolation, which can further exacerbate the pain experience.

On the other hand, mental health issues such as stress, anxiety, and depression can also contribute to the perception and intensity of pain. Stress can trigger the release of cortisol, a hormone that can increase inflammation and amplify pain signals in the body. Anxiety and depression can lower pain tolerance and make it harder to cope with pain daily.

Individuals with chronic pain need to address their mental health to effectively manage their pain. Therapies such as cognitive-behavioral therapy (CBT) have been proven to be effective in helping individuals cope with both pain and mental health issues. By identifying and challenging negative thought patterns, individuals can learn to better manage their pain and improve their overall quality of life.

Techniques for Managing Stress and Anxiety Related to Chronic Pain

Managing stress and anxiety related to chronic pain is crucial for alleviating pain and improving overall well-being. One effective technique for managing stress and anxiety is relaxation techniques such as deep breathing, progressive muscle relaxation, and guided imagery. These techniques help calm the nervous system and reduce the perception of pain.

Mindfulness practices have also been shown to be effective in managing stress, anxiety, and pain. Mindfulness involves paying attention to the present moment without judgment, which can help individuals develop a greater sense of control over their thoughts and emotions. Mindful practices such as meditation, yoga, and tai chi can help individuals cultivate a sense of calm and improve their ability to cope with pain.

Additionally, engaging in regular physical activity can help reduce stress and anxiety, improve mood, and alleviate pain. Exercise releases endorphins, which are natural painkillers produced by the body. It also helps improve flexibility, strength, and overall physical function, which can decrease the perception of pain and improve quality of life.

Incorporating relaxation techniques, mindfulness practices, and regular physical activity into daily life can help individuals better manage stress and anxiety related to chronic pain. By addressing mental health issues and developing healthy coping mechanisms, individuals can improve their overall well-being and enhance their ability to effectively manage their pain.

In conclusion, the mind-body connection plays a crucial role in the experience of chronic pain. Understanding the link between mental health and pain, as well as learning techniques for managing stress and anxiety, can greatly improve an individual's quality of life. By incorporating relaxation techniques, mindfulness practices, and regular physical activity into daily life, individuals can better cope with pain and improve their overall well-being.

7

Chapter 7: Creating a Holistic Pain Management Plan

Living with chronic pain can be overwhelming and debilitating, impacting every aspect of your life. While traditional medical treatments can be effective for managing pain, they often come with unwanted side effects and limitations. This is why many individuals are turning to holistic approaches to pain management, which focus on treating the whole person - mind, body, and spirit.

Creating a personalized pain management plan is essential for finding relief that works for you. This plan should take into consideration your individual needs, preferences, and goals. By working with a holistic practitioner, you can develop a comprehensive approach to managing your pain that goes beyond just treating the symptoms.

One of the first steps in creating a holistic pain management plan is setting realistic goals for pain relief and overall wellness. It's important to understand that managing chronic pain is a journey, and it may take time to find the right combination of treatments that work for you. Setting achievable goals can help you stay motivated and track your progress along the way.

When setting goals for pain relief, it's important to be specific and measurable. For example, instead of saying you want to "reduce pain," you could set a goal of "decreasing pain levels by 20% within the next three months." This allows you to track your progress and adjust your treatment plan as needed.

In addition to pain relief, it's also important to focus on your overall wellness. This can include improving your physical fitness, managing stress, getting enough sleep, and maintaining a healthy diet. By addressing these areas, you can help support your body's natural healing processes and reduce inflammation, which can contribute to pain.

To help you create a holistic pain management plan, there are a variety of resources available to you. One option is to seek out holistic practitioners who specialize in treating chronic pain. These practitioners may include acupuncturists, chiropractors, massage therapists, naturopathic doctors, and more. By working with a team of holistic healthcare providers, you can receive comprehensive care that addresses your physical, emotional, and spiritual needs.

Another resource for finding support in managing chronic pain is to join a support group. Support groups can provide you with a sense of community, connection, and understanding from others who are going through similar experiences. This can be invaluable in helping you cope with the challenges of living with chronic pain and finding inspiration and motivation to continue your healing journey.

As you work to create a holistic pain management plan, it's important to remember that there is no one-size-fits-all approach to managing chronic pain. What works for one person may not work for another, so it's important to listen to your body and be open to trying different treatments and therapies until you find what works best for you.

In conclusion, creating a holistic pain management plan involves setting realistic goals for pain relief and overall wellness, finding holistic practitioners who can support your healing journey, and connecting with support groups for additional encouragement and understanding. By taking a comprehensive approach to manage your pain, you can improve your quality of life and find relief that works for you.

8

Chapter 8: Alternative Therapies for Chronic Pain

Chronic pain affects millions of people worldwide and can significantly impact their quality of life. While traditional pain management approaches such as medication and physical therapy can be effective, some individuals may seek alternative therapies to help alleviate their symptoms. In this chapter, we will explore lesser-known alternative therapies such as biofeedback, hydrotherapy, and aromatherapy, and discuss their potential benefits for individuals living with chronic pain.

Exploration of Lesser-Known Alternative Therapies

Biofeedback is a mind-body technique that teaches individuals how to control physiological processes such as muscle tension and heart rate through feedback from electronic sensors. By learning to manipulate these processes, individuals can reduce their experience of pain and improve their overall well-being. Research has shown that biofeedback can be effective in managing chronic pain conditions such as migraines, fibromyalgia, and lower back pain.

Hydrotherapy, also known as water therapy, involves the use of water in various forms such as baths, pools, and saunas to help reduce pain and promote relaxation. The buoyancy of water can reduce pressure on the joints and muscles, making it an ideal therapy for individuals with conditions such as arthritis and chronic back pain. Hydrotherapy can also improve circulation and flexibility, leading to decreased pain and improved mobility.

Aromatherapy utilizes the therapeutic properties of essential oils derived from plants to promote relaxation, reduce stress, and alleviate pain. When inhaled or applied to the skin, these oils can have a powerful impact on the body and mind. Certain essential oils such as lavender, peppermint, and eucalyptus have analgesic and anti-inflammatory properties that can help reduce pain and inflammation in individuals with chronic pain conditions.

Case Studies Highlighting the Effectiveness of Alternative Treatments

In a recent study, a group of individuals with chronic migraines underwent biofeedback training over twelve weeks. By learning to control their muscle tension and heart rate, participants reported a significant decrease in the frequency and intensity of their migraines, as well as improvements in their overall quality of life. These findings suggest that biofeedback can be a valuable tool in managing chronic pain conditions.

Another study examined the effects of hydrotherapy on individuals with osteoarthritis of the knee. Participants who engaged in regular hydrotherapy sessions experienced a reduction in pain and stiffness, as well as improvements in their physical function and quality of life. These results demonstrate the potential benefits of hydrotherapy as a complementary treatment for individuals with chronic joint pain.

Considerations for Integrating Alternative Therapies into a Pain Management Regimen

When considering alternative therapies for chronic pain, it is important to consult with a healthcare provider to ensure that the chosen treatment is safe and appropriate for individual needs. Integrating alternative therapies into a pain management regimen can provide a holistic approach to pain relief and improve overall well-being.

It is also essential to approach alternative therapies with an open mind and a willingness to explore different treatment options. By incorporating biofeedback, hydrotherapy, or aromatherapy into a pain management regimen, individuals may discover new ways to manage their symptoms and improve their quality of life.

In conclusion, alternative therapies such as biofeedback, hydrotherapy, and aromatherapy can offer individuals living with chronic pain additional tools to manage their symptoms and improve their overall well-being. By exploring these lesser-known therapies and considering their potential benefits, individuals can enhance their pain management regimen and find relief from their symptoms.

9

Chapter 9: Sleep and Chronic Pain

Sleep is a crucial aspect of our overall health and well-being, playing a significant role in our ability to manage chronic pain. The impact of sleep quality on chronic pain cannot be overstated, as inadequate rest can exacerbate pain symptoms and hinder our ability to effectively cope with them. In this chapter, we will explore the relationship between sleep and chronic pain, as well as strategies for improving sleep hygiene and managing insomnia to promote pain relief and overall well-being.

The Impact of Sleep Quality on Chronic Pain

Research has consistently shown that poor sleep quality is strongly associated with increased pain sensitivity and intensity in individuals with chronic pain conditions. When we do not get enough quality sleep, our bodies become more sensitive to pain signals, making us more susceptible to experiencing heightened pain levels. Additionally, sleep deprivation can worsen inflammation and impair the body's ability to recover from injury or illness, further contributing to the cycle of pain.

Furthermore, the relationship between sleep and pain is bidirectional, meaning that chronic pain can also disrupt sleep patterns and lead to insomnia or other sleep disturbances. This creates a vicious cycle where poor sleep exacerbates pain, which in turn disrupts sleep, perpetuating the cycle of pain and sleep disturbances.

Strategies for Improving Sleep Hygiene and Managing Insomnia

To break the cycle of pain and poor sleep, it is essential to prioritize good sleep hygiene and develop strategies for managing insomnia. Some effective strategies for improving sleep quality and promoting restful sleep include:

Establishing a consistent sleep schedule: Go to bed and wake up at the same time every day, even on weekends, to regulate your body's internal clock and promote a healthy sleep-wake cycle.

Creating a calming bedtime routine: Engage in relaxing activities before bed, such as reading a book, taking a warm bath, or practicing mindfulness meditation, to signal to your body that it is time to wind down and prepare for sleep.

Creating a comfortable sleep environment: Ensure that your bedroom is conducive to sleep by keeping it cool, dark, and quiet, and investing in a comfortable mattress and pillows to support restful sleep.

Limiting caffeine and alcohol intake: Avoid consuming stimulants like caffeine and alcohol close to bedtime, as they can disrupt sleep patterns and inhibit your ability to fall asleep and stay asleep.

Practicing relaxation techniques: Incorporate relaxation techniques such as deep breathing exercises, progressive muscle relaxation, or guided imagery to calm your mind and body and promote restful sleep.

How Adequate Rest Contributes to Overall Pain Relief and Well-being

Adequate rest is essential for promoting pain relief and overall well-being in individuals with chronic pain. When we prioritize good sleep hygiene and ensure that we are getting enough quality rest, we are better equipped to manage pain symptoms and improve our overall quality of life. Restful sleep allows our bodies to repair and regenerate, reducing inflammation, boosting immune function, and facilitating the healing process.

Furthermore, adequate rest can have a positive impact on mood, cognitive function, and overall mental health, making it easier to cope with pain and maintain a positive outlook on life. By prioritizing sleep and implementing strategies for improving sleep quality, individuals with chronic pain can experience significant improvements in their pain symptoms and overall well-being.

In conclusion, sleep plays a critical role in the management of chronic pain, with the quality of rest directly impacting pain sensitivity and intensity. By prioritizing good sleep hygiene, managing insomnia, and ensuring that we are getting enough quality rest, individuals with chronic pain can experience significant improvements in their pain symptoms and overall well-being. It is essential to recognize the importance of sleep in the management of chronic pain and take proactive steps to promote restful sleep for optimal pain relief and overall health.

10

Chapter 10: Technology and Chronic Pain Management

Chronic pain affects millions of individuals worldwide, impacting their daily lives and overall well-being. Traditionally, pain management has relied on medications, physical therapy, and other conventional treatments. However, in recent years, technological advancements have revolutionized the field of chronic pain management, offering new and innovative solutions for those suffering from persistent pain. In this chapter, we will explore the role of technology in enhancing traditional and holistic approaches to pain relief, as well as provide practical tips for utilizing technology for chronic pain management.

Overview of Technological Advancements in Pain Management

One of the most significant technological advancements in chronic pain management is the development of wearable devices. These devices, such as smartwatches and fitness trackers, can monitor various aspects of an individual's health, including heart rate, sleep patterns, and physical activity levels.

In the context of chronic pain, wearable devices can track pain levels and provide real-time feedback on how certain activities or interventions may be affecting pain levels.

Virtual reality (VR) is another technology that has shown promising results in pain management. By immersing individuals in a virtual environment, VR can distract the brain from focusing on pain signals, providing temporary relief. Additionally, VR can be used in combination with traditional therapies, such as physical therapy, to enhance pain relief and improve outcomes.

Medicine has also emerged as a valuable tool in chronic pain management, particularly in remote or underserved areas where access to healthcare providers may be limited. Through medicine platforms, individuals can consult with healthcare professionals, receive personalized treatment plans, and access resources for managing their pain from the comfort of their own homes.

How Technology Can Enhance Traditional and Holistic Approaches to Pain Relief

Technology has the potential to enhance traditional and holistic approaches to pain relief by providing individuals with greater control over their pain management strategies. For example, wearable devices can help individuals track their activity levels and identify patterns that may exacerbate their pain, empowering them to make informed decisions about their lifestyle choices.

Virtual reality can be used as a complementary therapy to traditional pain management techniques, such as medication and physical therapy. By incorporating VR into a comprehensive treatment plan, individuals may experience greater pain relief and improved quality of life.

Telemedicine can bridge the gap between individuals and healthcare providers, allowing for more frequent communication and monitoring of pain management strategies. Through telemedicine platforms, individuals can receive ongoing support and guidance from healthcare professionals, leading to more effective pain management outcomes.

Practical Tips for Utilizing Technology for Chronic Pain Management

When utilizing technology for chronic pain management, it is important to approach it with a proactive and informed mindset. Here are some practical tips for incorporating technology into your pain management routine:

Research and explore different types of wearable devices and virtual reality programs to find the ones that best suit your needs and preferences.

Work closely with your healthcare provider to develop a comprehensive pain management plan that incorporates both traditional and technological interventions.

Use wearable devices to track your pain levels, activity levels, and sleep patterns, and share this information with your healthcare provider to inform your treatment plan.

Incorporate virtual reality into your pain management routine by using VR programs during times of increased pain or discomfort.

Utilize medicine platforms to connect with healthcare providers, ask questions, and receive ongoing support and guidance for managing your chronic pain.

By embracing technology as a complement to traditional and holistic approaches to pain relief, individuals can take greater control of their chronic pain management journey and experience improved outcomes.

11

Chapter 11: Herbal Remedies and Supplements for Pain Relief

Exploration of herbal remedies and supplements known for their pain-relieving properties

Throughout history, herbal remedies and supplements have been used for their pain-relieving properties. From traditional Chinese medicine to Ayurvedic practices, various plants and herbs have been prized for their ability to alleviate pain. In recent years, there has been a resurgence of interest in natural remedies as people seek alternatives to conventional pharmaceuticals. Here, we will explore some of the most popular herbal remedies and supplements known for their pain-relieving properties.

One of the most well-known herbal remedies for pain relief is turmeric. This bright yellow spice has been used in traditional Indian medicine for centuries and has gained popularity in the West for its potent anti-inflammatory properties. Curcumin, the active compound in turmeric, has been shown to reduce pain and inflammation in conditions such as arthritis and fibrillation. Turmeric can be consumed in its natural form or taken as a supplement for more concentrated benefits.

Another popular herbal remedy for pain relief is ginger. This spicy root has long been used in traditional medicine for its anti-inflammatory and analgesic properties. Ginger can be consumed fresh, dried, or in supplement form to help alleviate pain from conditions such as osteoarthritis and muscle soreness. Some studies have even shown ginger to be as effective as anti-inflammatory drugs (NSAIDs) in reducing pain and inflammation.

Devil's Claw is another herb known for its pain-relieving properties. Native to southern Africa, devil's claw has been traditionally used to treat arthritis, back pain, and other inflammatory conditions. Studies have shown that devil's claw can help reduce pain and improve mobility in individuals with osteoarthritis. Devil's claw can be taken as a supplement or brewed into a tea for natural pain relief.

Safety considerations and potential interactions with medications

While herbal remedies and supplements can be effective for pain relief, it is important to consider safety considerations and potential interactions with medications. Just because a remedy is natural does not mean it is always safe, especially when taken in high doses or combination with other medications. It is important to consult with a healthcare professional before incorporating herbs and supplements into your pain management plan.

Some herbs and supplements may interact with medications, either enhancing or inhibiting their effects. For example, St. John's Wort, a popular herbal remedy for depression, can interact with certain medications used for pain management, such as opioids and antidepressants. Similarly, turmeric supplements can interact with blood thinners and increase the risk of bleeding. It is important to disclose all herbs and supplements you are taking to your healthcare provider to avoid potential drug interactions.

Guidance on incorporating herbs and supplements into a comprehensive pain management plan.

When incorporating herbs and supplements into a comprehensive pain management plan, it is important to approach it holistically. Herbal remedies and supplements should not be used as a standalone treatment but rather as part of a multi-faceted approach to pain relief. Here are some tips for integrating herbs and supplements into your pain management plan:

Consult with a healthcare professional: Before starting any herbal remedy or supplement, consult with a healthcare provider to ensure it is safe and appropriate for your condition.

Start with low doses: Begin with a low dose of the herb or supplement and gradually increase as needed. Monitor for any adverse effects or interactions with medications.

Be consistent: Herbal remedies and supplements may take time to build up in your system and show results. Be consistent with your dosing and give it time to work.

Keep a journal: Keep track of your pain levels, symptoms, and the effects of the herbs and supplements you are taking. This can help you and your healthcare provider assess the effectiveness of the treatment.

In conclusion, herbal remedies and supplements can be valuable additions to a comprehensive pain management plan. When used safely and effectively, herbs and supplements can provide natural pain relief and reduce the need for conventional medications. By exploring different herbal remedies, considering safety considerations, and integrating them into a holistic pain management plan, individuals can take control of their pain and improve their quality of life.

12

Chapter 12: Support Systems for Coping with Chronic Pain

Living with chronic pain can be an isolating and challenging experience. The physical and emotional toll it takes on individuals can be overwhelming, making it crucial to have a strong support system in place. Research has shown that social support plays a vital role in managing chronic pain, helping individuals cope with daily struggles, and improving their overall quality of life.

Importance of Social Support in Managing Chronic Pain

Social support refers to the network of family, friends, and peers who provide emotional, practical, and informational assistance during difficult times. When it comes to chronic pain, having a supportive network can make a significant difference in how individuals cope with their condition. Studies have shown that individuals who have strong social support systems tend to experience less pain, have better psychological well-being, and are more likely to adhere to treatment regimens.

Types of Support Systems Available

Family and Friends: Family members and close friends can be a valuable source of support for individuals living with chronic pain. They can provide emotional support, help with daily tasks, and offer companionship during tough times. Individuals need to communicate their needs and boundaries to their loved ones, ensuring that they understand the challenges they are facing and how they can best support them.

Support Groups: Support groups can also be an effective way for individuals to connect with others who are going through similar experiences. These groups provide a safe space for individuals to share their struggles, offer empathy and understanding, and learn coping strategies from others who are facing similar challenges. Joining a support group can help individuals feel less alone in their pain and provide a sense of community and belonging.

Tips for Effectively Communicating Pain-Related Needs and Boundaries

Effective communication is key to building and maintaining a strong support system. When communicating with family, friends, or support group members about your chronic pain, consider the following tips:

Be open and honest: Share your experiences, feelings, and needs openly with your support system. This can help them better understand what you are going through and how they can best support you.

Set boundaries: It is important to set boundaries with your support system to ensure that your needs are being met without feeling overwhelmed or burdened. Let them know what you are comfortable with and what you need from them.

Be specific: Communicate your pain-related needs to your support system. Whether it is help with household tasks, emotional support, or simply someone to listen, be specific about how they can best assist you.

Express gratitude: Show appreciation for the support you receive from your loved ones and support group members. Gratitude can strengthen your relationships and motivate them to continue supporting you.

In conclusion, having a strong support system is essential for individuals living with chronic pain. Whether it is family, friends, or support groups, having a network of people who understand your struggles and provide emotional, practical, and informational support can make a significant difference in how you manage your pain. By effectively communicating your pain-related needs and boundaries to your support system, you can build stronger relationships and improve your overall quality of life.

13

Chapter 13: Lifestyle Modifications for Pain Management

Chronic pain is a complex and multifaceted condition that can be influenced by a variety of lifestyle factors. Identifying and addressing these factors is crucial in effectively managing pain and improving overall quality of life. In this chapter, we will discuss the importance of ergonomics, posture, and smoking cessation in pain management, as well as strategies for making sustainable lifestyle changes to alleviate pain symptoms and incorporating self-care practices into daily life for long-term pain management.

Ergonomics and Posture

Ergonomics and posture play a significant role in the development and exacerbation of chronic pain. Poor ergonomic practices, such as improper workstation setup or lifting techniques, can lead to musculoskeletal imbalances and contribute to pain in the neck, back, shoulders, and other areas of the body. Similarly, poor posture can place unnecessary strain on the muscles and joints, leading to discomfort and pain over time.

To improve ergonomics and posture and reduce the risk of pain, it is important to make simple adjustments to your daily routine. This may include using ergonomic office furniture, adjusting the height of your computer monitor and chair, practicing proper lifting techniques, and taking regular breaks to stretch and move throughout the day. Additionally, incorporating exercises that strengthen the core and improve flexibility can help support proper posture and reduce the risk of pain.

Smoking Cessation

Smoking is a well-known risk factor for chronic pain, as it can contribute to inflammation, decreased blood flow, and impaired healing processes in the body. Quitting smoking is not only important for improving overall health and reducing the risk of chronic diseases, but it can also help alleviate pain symptoms and improve the effectiveness of pain management strategies.

If you smoke and experience chronic pain, it is important to seek support and resources to help you quit. This may include talking to your healthcare provider, joining a smoking cessation program, using nicotine replacement therapy, or exploring alternative therapies such as acupuncture or mindfulness-based practices. By quitting smoking, you can reduce inflammation in the body, improve circulation, and support the body's natural healing processes, leading to reduced pain and improved quality of life.

Sustainable Lifestyle Changes

Making sustainable lifestyle changes is essential for long-term pain management and overall well-being. While it may be tempting to rely on quick fixes or temporary solutions, true relief from chronic pain requires a comprehensive approach that addresses the underlying causes of pain and supports the body's natural healing processes.

To make sustainable lifestyle changes, it is important to set realistic goals, prioritize self-care practices, and enlist the support of healthcare providers, therapists, and other professionals as needed. This may include incorporating regular exercise, practicing stress management techniques, improving sleep quality, and maintaining a healthy diet rich in anti-inflammatory foods. By making small, gradual changes to your daily routine, you can create lasting improvements in pain symptoms and overall quality of life.

Self-Care Practices

Incorporating self-care practices into your daily routine is essential for long-term pain management and overall well-being. Self-care practices can help reduce stress, improve mood, and support the body's natural healing processes, leading to reduced pain and improved quality of life.

Some self-care practices that may help alleviate pain symptoms include mindfulness meditation, deep breathing exercises, progressive muscle relaxation, gentle yoga, and warm baths or showers. Additionally, activities that promote relaxation and stress reduction, such as spending time in nature, listening to music, or engaging in creative pursuits, can help support overall well-being and reduce pain levels.

By incorporating self-care practices into your daily life, you can create a supportive and nurturing environment that promotes healing and reduces the impact of chronic pain on your physical, emotional, and mental well-being.

In conclusion, lifestyle modifications play a crucial role in pain management and overall well-being. By identifying and addressing factors such as ergonomics, posture, and smoking cessation, making sustainable lifestyle changes, and incorporating self-care practices into your daily routine, you can effectively manage chronic pain and improve your quality of life. Take the time to prioritize your health and well-being, and you will reap the benefits of reduced pain, increased mobility, and enhanced overall wellness.

14

Chapter 14: Spirituality and Chronic Pain

Chronic pain is a complex and challenging condition that affects millions of people around the world. It can have a profound impact on all aspects of a person's life, including their physical, emotional, and spiritual well-being. In recent years, there has been growing interest in the role of spirituality in coping with chronic pain, as many individuals seek alternative ways to find peace and comfort amidst their suffering.

Exploration of the role of spirituality in coping with chronic pain

Spirituality can be defined as a deeply personal belief system that provides individuals with a sense of purpose, meaning, and connection to something greater than themselves. For many people, spirituality plays a significant role in how they navigate the challenges of chronic pain. By tapping into their spiritual beliefs, individuals can find strength, resilience, and hope in their suffering.

One of the key ways in which spirituality can help individuals cope with chronic pain is by providing a sense of perspective and purpose. When faced with the overwhelming and constant presence of pain, it can be easy to feel lost, hopeless, and disconnected from the world around us. However, by turning to our spiritual beliefs, we can find meaning in our suffering and see it as an opportunity for growth, healing, and transformation.

Practices such as prayer, meditation, and mindfulness for finding peace midst pain.

Prayer, meditation, and mindfulness are powerful tools that can help individuals find peace and comfort midst the challenges of chronic pain. These practices have been used for centuries by people of all faith traditions to help them connect with their inner selves, cultivate a sense of calm and tranquility, and find solace in times of distress.

Prayer is a deeply personal and intimate conversation with a higher power, whether that be God, the universe, or a spiritual guide. Through prayer, individuals can express their fears, hopes, and desires, and seek guidance, support, and healing in the face of their pain.

Meditation is a practice that involves focusing the mind on the present moment, cultivating awareness and acceptance of one's thoughts, emotions, and physical sensations. By practicing meditation, individuals can learn to observe their pain without judgment or resistance and find a sense of peace and serenity midst their suffering.

Mindfulness is a way of living in which individuals strive to be fully present and engaged in each moment, paying attention to their thoughts, feelings, and sensations without being overwhelmed by them. By practicing mindfulness, individuals can learn to accept their pain with compassion and self-compassion and find resilience and strength in the face of their suffering.

How spiritual beliefs can provide comfort and resilience in the face of suffering.

Spiritual beliefs can provide individuals with comfort, solace, and resilience in the face of chronic pain. By drawing on their faith, individuals can find a sense of peace, hope, and acceptance in their suffering. Whether it be through prayer, meditation, or mindfulness, spiritual practices can help individuals connect with their inner selves, cultivate a sense of gratitude and grace, and find strength and courage to face their pain with dignity and grace.

In conclusion, spirituality can play a powerful and transformative role in how individuals cope with chronic pain. By exploring their spiritual beliefs, practicing prayer, meditation, and mindfulness, and finding comfort and resilience in the face of suffering, individuals can find peace, healing, and hope midst their pain.

15

Chapter 15: Advocacy and Empowerment in Pain Management

Advocacy and empowerment play crucial roles in navigating the complex world of pain management. Individuals living with chronic pain often face barriers to accessing effective treatment and support, and advocating for oneself can make a significant difference in the quality of care received. In this chapter, we will explore the importance of self-advocacy in the healthcare system, strategies for navigating medical appointments, insurance, and treatment options, and how to empower individuals with chronic pain to become active participants in their care.

The Importance of Advocating for Oneself in the Healthcare System

Advocating for oneself in the healthcare system is essential for individuals living with chronic pain. Many people with chronic pain face challenges such as stigma, lack of understanding from healthcare providers, and difficulty accessing appropriate treatment. By advocating for oneself, individuals can ensure that their voices are heard, and their needs are met.

One of the first steps in advocating for oneself is to educate oneself about chronic pain and available treatment options. This includes researching different types of pain management techniques, understanding the potential side effects of medications, and learning about alternative therapies. Armed with this knowledge, individuals can have more informed discussions with their healthcare providers and make better decisions about their care.

Another important aspect of self-advocacy is assertiveness. Individuals must speak up about their pain levels, treatment preferences, and any concerns they may have. This can help ensure that healthcare providers take their symptoms seriously and tailor treatment plans to meet their specific needs.

Strategies for Navigating Medical Appointments, Insurance, and Treatment Options

Navigating medical appointments, insurance, and treatment options can be overwhelming for individuals living with chronic pain. However, some strategies can help make this process easier and more manageable.

One strategy is to come prepared for medical appointments. This includes bringing a list of symptoms, questions, and concerns to discuss with the healthcare provider. It can also be helpful to keep a pain journal to track symptoms and treatment outcomes, which can provide valuable information for the healthcare provider.

Another important aspect of navigating medical appointments is communication. Individuals should feel comfortable discussing their pain levels, treatment preferences, and any concerns they may have. It is also important to ask questions if something is unclear and to advocate for oneself if necessary.

When it comes to insurance and treatment options, individuals should be proactive in researching coverage options and advocating for the treatments that are most effective for them. This may involve working with healthcare providers to submit prior authorization requests, appealing denials of coverage, or exploring alternative treatment options.

Empowering Individuals with Chronic Pain to Become Active Participants in Their Care

Empowering individuals with chronic pain to become active participants in their care is essential for improving treatment outcomes and quality of life. One way to empower individuals is to involve them in decision-making processes about their care. This can include discussing treatment options, setting goals for pain management, and creating personalized treatment plans.

Education is another key component of empowerment. By educating individuals about their condition, treatment options, and self-management strategies, they can make more informed decisions about their care and feel more confident in managing their pain.

Support is also important for empowering individuals with chronic pain. This may involve connecting with peer support groups, participating in counseling or therapy, or working with healthcare providers who understand and validate their experiences.

In conclusion, advocacy and empowerment are essential components of effective pain management. By advocating for oneself in the healthcare system, navigating medical appointments, insurance, and treatment options, and empowering individuals with chronic pain to become active participants in their care, individuals can take control of their pain management journey and improve their quality of life.

16

Chapter 16: Long-Term Strategies for Maintaining Pain Relief

As you continue your journey toward managing chronic pain, it is crucial to develop long-term strategies to sustain progress and prevent pain flare-ups over time. While it may seem daunting, with dedication and perseverance, you can find relief and improve your quality of life. In this chapter, we will discuss tips for maintaining pain relief, the importance of ongoing self-assessment and adaptation of pain management strategies, and the encouragement to remain resilient and hopeful on your path to wellness.

Tips for Sustaining Progress and Preventing Pain Flare-Ups Over Time

To maintain pain relief over the long term, it is essential to incorporate healthy habits into your daily routine. Here are some tips to help you sustain progress and prevent pain flare-ups:

Stay active: Regular exercise is key to managing chronic pain. Find activities that you enjoy and are gentle on your body, such as walking, swimming, or yoga. Physical activity can help strengthen muscles, improve flexibility, and release feel-good endorphins that can help alleviate pain.

Practice good posture: Poor posture can put a strain on your muscles and joints, leading to increased pain. Be mindful of your posture throughout the day, whether sitting, standing, or walking. Consider using ergonomic furniture or tools to support proper alignment.

Manage stress: Stress can exacerbate pain and make it harder to find relief. Practice relaxation techniques such as deep breathing, meditation, or mindfulness to help reduce stress levels. Prioritize self-care activities that bring you joy and relaxation.

Get enough rest: Adequate sleep is essential for managing chronic pain. Aim for 7-9 hours of quality sleep each night to support your body's healing and recovery processes. Create a calming bedtime routine and establish a comfortable sleep environment to promote restful sleep.

Maintain a healthy diet: Eating a balanced diet rich in fruits, vegetables, whole grains, and lean proteins can help reduce inflammation and support overall health. Stay hydrated and limit your consumption of processed foods, sugar, and caffeine, which can exacerbate pain.

The Importance of Ongoing Self-Assessment and Adaptation of

Pain Management Strategies

Managing chronic pain is a dynamic process that requires continuous self-assessment and adaptation of pain management strategies. As you navigate your journey, pay attention to how your body responds to treatments and interventions. Keep a pain journal to track your symptoms, triggers, and progress over time. Be open to trying new approaches and adjusting your plan as needed to find what works best for you.

Consult with your healthcare team regularly to discuss your pain management goals and any changes in your condition. They can provide guidance, support, and expertise to help you optimize your treatment plan. Be proactive in advocating for your needs and seeking out additional resources or therapies that may benefit you.

Encouragement to Remain Resilient and Hopeful on the Journey Toward Wellness

Living with chronic pain can be challenging, but it is important to remain resilient and hopeful on your path to wellness. Embrace a positive mindset and believe in your ability to overcome obstacles and achieve your goals. Surround yourself with a supportive network of family, friends, and healthcare professionals who understand and encourage your journey.

Celebrate your successes, no matter how small, and acknowledge the progress you have made. Stay focused on the present moment and practice gratitude for the blessings in your life. Remember that healing is a gradual process, and setbacks are a natural part of the journey. Stay committed to your self-care routine and trust in your ability to navigate through challenges with strength and determination.

In conclusion, maintaining pain relief over the long term requires dedication, resilience, and a willingness to adapt. By incorporating healthy habits, practicing ongoing self-assessment, and staying hopeful on your journey toward wellness, you can find relief and improve your quality of life. Stay committed to your self-care routine and believe in your ability to thrive despite chronic pain.

17

Chapter 17: Coping Techniques for Flare-Ups and Setbacks

Dealing with chronic pain can be a challenging and often unpredictable journey. Despite our best efforts to manage our symptoms, there may be times when flare-ups occur, causing a sudden increase in pain intensity and making it difficult to carry out daily activities. In these moments, it is important to have coping strategies in place to help navigate through the pain and emotional challenges that may arise.

Strategies for Managing Sudden Increases in Pain Intensity

When faced with a flare-up, it is crucial to have a plan in place to help manage the sudden increase in pain intensity. One effective strategy is to practice deep breathing exercises, which can help relax the body and distract from the pain. Additionally, using heat or cold therapy, such as a heating pad or ice pack, can provide relief by reducing inflammation and numbing the area of pain.

Engaging in gentle stretching or low-impact exercises, such as yoga or tai chi, can also help to alleviate pain and improve flexibility. It is important to listen to your body and avoid overexerting yourself during a flare-up, as this can potentially worsen symptoms.

If the pain becomes overwhelming, it may be helpful to utilize distraction techniques, such as listening to music, watching a movie, or practicing mindfulness meditation. These activities can help shift focus away from the pain and promote relaxation.

Tips for Navigating Emotional Challenges During Flare-Ups

In addition to managing physical pain, it is important to address the emotional challenges that may accompany flare-ups. Feelings of frustration, anger, and helplessness are common during these times, and it is essential to acknowledge and validate these emotions.

One helpful tip is to practice self-compassion and be kind to yourself during flare-ups. Remind yourself that it is okay to feel frustrated or upset and that these emotions are a natural response to living with chronic pain. Seeking support from loved ones, a therapist, or a support group can also be beneficial in processing these emotions and finding ways to cope.

Creating a Personalized Action Plan for Coping with Setbacks

To effectively navigate through flare-ups and setbacks, it is important to create a personalized action plan that outlines strategies for managing symptoms and addressing emotional challenges. This plan should be tailored to your individual needs and preferences, considering what has worked well for you in the past.

Start by identifying specific coping techniques that have been effective in managing pain, such as relaxation exercises, physical therapy, or medication. Create a list of resources and contacts, including healthcare providers, therapists, and support groups, that you can reach out to for assistance during flare-ups.

Develop a routine for self-care that includes regular exercise, healthy eating, adequate sleep, and stress management techniques. Prioritize activities that bring you joy and relaxation, such as spending time with loved ones, engaging in hobbies, or practicing mindfulness.

Incorporate strategies for managing emotional challenges, such as journaling, practicing gratitude, or seeking professional counseling when needed. Remember that it is okay to ask for help and support from others and that you do not have to navigate through setbacks alone.

By creating a personalized action plan for coping with flare-ups and setbacks, you can empower yourself to effectively manage symptoms, address emotional challenges, and continue moving forward on your journey toward healing and well-being.

18

Chapter 18: Exploring Energy Healing Modalities for Pain Relief

Introduction

Energy healing modalities have been gaining popularity in recent years as complementary therapies for pain relief. These practices, which focus on restoring the body's natural energy flow, can be effective in managing chronic pain and promoting overall well-being. In this chapter, we will explore two prominent energy-based therapies, Reiki and Qigong, and discuss their principles, effects on pain, and practical techniques for incorporating them into a comprehensive pain management approach.

Understanding the Principles behind Energy Healing

Reiki is a Japanese technique that involves the laying on of hands to channel energy to promote healing and relaxation. The practitioner acts as a conduit for universal life force energy, which is believed to flow through the body and support its natural ability to heal. Reiki sessions can help balance the body's energy center or chakras and release blockages that may be contributing to pain and discomfort.

Qigong, on the other hand, is a Chinese practice that combines movement, breathwork, and meditation to cultivate and balance the body's vital energy, or Qi. Through gentle exercises and focused intention, practitioners can strengthen their Qi and promote healing on physical, emotional, and spiritual levels. Qigong is often used to alleviate pain, reduce stress, and improve overall health and well-being.

Effects of Energy Healing on Pain

Both Reiki and Qigong are effective in relieving pain and promoting relaxation. Studies have demonstrated that these energy-healing modalities can reduce pain intensity and improve the quality of life for individuals with chronic conditions such as fibromyalgia, arthritis, and cancer. By restoring balance to the body's energy systems, Reiki and Qigong can help alleviate physical discomfort, reduce inflammation, and support the body's natural healing processes.

Practical Techniques for Incorporating Energy Healing

Incorporating Reiki and Qigong into a comprehensive pain management approach can enhance the effectiveness of conventional treatments and provide holistic support for individuals experiencing chronic pain. Practitioners can work with clients to develop personalized energy healing plans that address their specific needs and goals.

For example, a Reiki practitioner may perform hands-on or distance healing sessions to help clients release pain and tension, balance their energy centers, and promote relaxation. Reiki can be integrated into massage therapy, acupuncture, or other bodywork modalities to enhance their effects and support the body's ability to heal.

Similarly, individuals can practice Qigong exercises at home or in a group setting to cultivate their Qi, balance their energy, and alleviate pain. Simple movements, such as flowing and stretching exercises, can help improve circulation, reduce inflammation, and release tension in the body. Regular Qigong practice can also enhance mindfulness, reduce stress, and support emotional well-being, which can be beneficial for managing chronic pain.

In conclusion, energy healing modalities such as Reiki and Qigong offer valuable tools for managing pain and promoting overall health and well-being. By understanding the principles behind these practices, exploring their effects on pain, and incorporating practical techniques into a comprehensive pain management approach, individuals can experience relief, relaxation, and enhanced healing on physical, emotional, and spiritual levels.

19

Chapter 19: Integrative Approaches to Pain Management Combining Eastern and Western Medicine

In recent years, there has been a growing recognition of the benefits of integrating practices from both Eastern and Western medical traditions in the treatment of chronic pain. While Western medicine often focuses on the use of pharmaceuticals and invasive procedures to manage pain, Eastern medicine offers a holistic approach that considers the mind, body, and spirit as interconnected and emphasizes the importance of balance and harmony for overall health and well-being. By combining the strengths of both approaches, patients can experience more comprehensive and effective pain management.

One of the primary benefits of integrating practices from both Eastern and Western medicine is the ability to address pain from multiple angles. While Western medicine may provide immediate relief through medications or surgeries, Eastern practices such as acupuncture, yoga, tai chi, and meditation can help to address the underlying causes of pain by promoting relaxation, reducing inflammation, and improving circulation. By incorporating these complementary therapies into a patient's treatment plan, healthcare providers can offer a more comprehensive and personalized approach to pain management.

For specific chronic pain conditions, there are a variety of integrative approaches that have shown promise in improving symptoms and enhancing quality of life. For example, acupuncture is effective in relieving pain associated with conditions such as fibromyalgia, osteoarthritis, and migraines. By stimulating specific points in the body, acupuncture can help to release tension, reduce inflammation, and improve the flow of energy, or qi, throughout the body.

Similarly, yoga and tai chi are beneficial for individuals with chronic back pain, arthritis, and other musculoskeletal conditions. These mind-body practices focus on gentle movements, breathing exercises, and mindfulness techniques that can help to improve flexibility, strength, and balance, while also promoting relaxation and reducing stress. By incorporating these practices into a patient's daily routine, they can experience long-term benefits for their physical and emotional well-being.

In addition to specific therapies, an integrative approach to pain management also emphasizes the importance of finding balance and harmony in all aspects of life. This may include addressing dietary habits, sleep patterns, exercise routines, and stress management techniques to support overall health and well-being. By taking a holistic approach to healing, patients can cultivate a sense of self-awareness and self-care that can enhance their resilience and coping skills in the face of chronic pain.

Ultimately, the goal of integrative approaches to pain management is to empower patients to take an active role in their healing journey. By combining the best practices from both Eastern and Western medicine, healthcare providers can offer a more personalized and comprehensive approach to pain management that addresses the unique needs and preferences of everyone. Through a holistic focus on balance and harmony, patients can experience improved pain relief, enhanced quality of life, and a greater sense of overall well-being.

20

Chapter 20: The Role of Sleep Hygiene in Chronic Pain Management

Sleep is a fundamental aspect of human health and well-being, playing a crucial role in restoring and rejuvenating the body. For individuals experiencing chronic pain, the relationship between sleep and pain perception is complex and interconnected. Research has shown that poor sleep quality can exacerbate pain symptoms, while effective sleep hygiene practices can help alleviate pain and improve overall quality of life.

Understanding the Connection between Sleep Quality and Pain Perception

The relationship between sleep quality and pain perception is bidirectional, with each influencing the other in a vicious cycle. Chronic pain can disrupt sleep patterns, leading to difficulties falling asleep, staying asleep, and achieving restorative sleep. In turn, poor sleep can lower pain thresholds, increase pain sensitivity, and exacerbate existing pain conditions. This cycle can create a detrimental feedback loop, where pain and sleep disturbances feed off each other, perpetuating a cycle of discomfort and distress.

Research has shown that sleep disturbances can alter the body's pain processing pathways, leading to increased pain perception and decreased pain tolerance. Factors such as sleep fragmentation reduced deep sleep stages, and disrupted circadian rhythms can contribute to heightened pain sensitivity and intensity. Furthermore, sleep deprivation can impair the body's ability to regulate inflammation and immune responses, further exacerbating pain symptoms in individuals with chronic pain conditions.

Tips for Improving Sleep Hygiene to Enhance Pain Relief

Improving sleep hygiene practices can help break the cycle of poor sleep and pain, leading to better pain management and overall well-being. Here are some strategies to enhance sleep hygiene and promote restorative sleep in individuals with chronic pain:

Establish a Consistent Sleep Schedule: Going to bed and waking up at the same time every day can help regulate the body's circadian rhythms and improve sleep quality. Consistency in sleep patterns can promote restful sleep and enhance pain relief.

Create a Relaxing Bedtime Routine: Engaging in calming activities before bedtime, such as reading, meditating, or taking a warm bath, can help signal the body that it is time to wind down and prepare for sleep. Avoiding stimulating activities, such as watching TV or using electronic devices, can also promote relaxation and improve sleep quality.

Optimize Sleep Environment: Creating a conducive sleep environment can enhance sleep quality and promote pain relief. Ensure your bedroom is dark, quiet, and cool, and invest in a comfortable mattress and pillows to support restful sleep.

Practice Good Sleep Hygiene: Adopting healthy sleep habits, such as avoiding caffeine and alcohol close to bedtime, limiting screen time, and maintaining a comfortable sleep temperature, can improve sleep quality and alleviate pain symptoms.

Developing a Bedtime Routine Tailored to Individual Needs and Preferences

Developing a personalized bedtime routine can help individuals with chronic pain optimize their sleep hygiene practices and enhance pain relief. Tailoring bedtime rituals to individual needs and preferences can promote relaxation, reduce stress, and improve sleep quality. Some individuals may find that incorporating mindfulness techniques, such as deep breathing or progressive muscle relaxation, can help ease pain and promote restful sleep. Others may benefit from herbal teas, aromatherapy, or light stretching exercises before bedtime to enhance relaxation and prepare the body for sleep.

In conclusion, the relationship between sleep hygiene and chronic pain management is significant and multifaceted. By understanding the connection between sleep quality and pain perception, implementing effective sleep hygiene practices, and developing a personalized bedtime routine, individuals with chronic pain can improve their sleep quality, alleviate pain symptoms, and enhance their overall quality of life. By prioritizing sleep hygiene and adopting healthy sleep habits, individuals can break the cycle of poor sleep and pain, leading to better pain management and improved well-being.

21

Chapter 21: Utilizing Cognitive-Behavioral Therapy for Pain Management

Overview of Cognitive-Behavioral Therapy (CBT) and Its Application in Pain Management

Cognitive-behavioral therapy (CBT) is a widely used and evidence-based approach to treating a variety of mental health conditions, including anxiety, depression, and PTSD. In recent years, CBT has also been shown to be effective in helping individuals manage chronic pain. The underlying principle of CBT is that our thoughts, feelings, and behaviors are interconnected and that by changing our thoughts and behaviors, we can change how we feel.

When it comes to pain management, CBT can be a powerful tool for helping individuals cope with the physical and emotional challenges that come with chronic pain. By identifying and challenging negative thought patterns related to pain, individuals can learn to reframe their thinking and develop more positive coping skills.

Identifying and Challenging Negative Thought Patterns Related to Pain

One of the key components of CBT for pain management is identifying and challenging negative thought patterns related to pain. This involves helping individuals recognize and change the way they think about their pain. For example, someone who experiences chronic back pain may have thoughts such as "I'll never be able to do the things I used to do" or "This pain will never go away." These negative thoughts can contribute to feelings of hopelessness and depression, which in turn can make the pain feel even worse.

Through CBT, individuals can learn to identify these negative thought patterns and challenge them with more realistic and positive thoughts. For example, instead of thinking "This pain will never go away," they might reframe it as "I can manage my pain by practicing relaxation techniques and staying active." By changing their thinking in this way, individuals can begin to feel more in control of their pain and develop a sense of hope for the future.

Practical Exercises and Techniques for Promoting Positive Coping Skills and Resilience

In addition to identifying and challenging negative thought patterns, CBT for pain management also involves teaching individuals practical exercises and techniques for promoting positive coping skills and resilience. These techniques can help individuals manage their pain more effectively and improve their overall quality of life.

One common technique used in CBT for pain management is relaxation training. This involves teaching individuals how to relax their muscles and calm their minds to reduce stress and tension, which can exacerbate pain. Techniques such as deep breathing, progressive muscle relaxation, and guided imagery can be particularly effective in helping individuals manage their pain.

Another important aspect of CBT for pain management is developing coping skills and resilience. This involves helping individuals build their ability to cope with pain and adversity healthily and deceptively. By learning to problem-solve, communicate effectively, and practice self-care, individuals can develop the skills they need to navigate the challenges of living with chronic pain.

Overall, CBT for pain management is a powerful and effective approach to helping individuals cope with chronic pain. By identifying and challenging negative thought patterns related to pain, as well as teaching practical exercises and techniques for promoting positive coping skills and resilience, individuals can learn to manage their pain more effectively and improve their quality of life.

22

Chapter 22: Art Therapy and Creative Expression in Pain Relief

Art therapy has been recognized as a powerful tool in managing chronic pain and promoting emotional healing. By engaging in creative activities, individuals can explore their emotions, reduce stress, and improve their overall well-being. In this chapter, we will delve into the therapeutic benefits of art and creative expression for pain relief, and how it can be utilized as an effective coping mechanism for those experiencing chronic pain.

Exploring the Therapeutic Benefits of Art and Creative Expression for Chronic Pain Management

Art therapy involves the use of artistic activities, such as drawing, painting, and sculpting, to help individuals express their emotions and thoughts in a non-verbal way. For those living with chronic pain, art therapy can provide a means of coping with the physical and emotional challenges they face daily. Through artistic expression, individuals can gain insight into their pain experience, and develop new ways of coping with their symptoms.

Research has shown that engaging in artistic activities can help reduce pain perception and improve overall quality of life for individuals with chronic pain. By focusing on the creative process, individuals can shift their attention away from their pain and engage in a positive and meaningful activity. This can lead to a reduction in stress levels, improved mood, and increased feelings of empowerment and control over their pain.

Engaging in Artistic Activities to Reduce Stress and Improve Mood

Creating art can be a therapeutic and cathartic experience for individuals living with chronic pain. By engaging in artistic activities, individuals can channel their emotions and express themselves in a safe and non-judgmental environment. This can help reduce stress levels, improve mood, and promote a sense of relaxation and well-being.

Artistic activities, such as drawing, painting, and collage-making, can also help individuals develop new coping strategies for managing their pain. Through the creative process, individuals can explore different ways of expressing their emotions and thoughts, and develop a greater sense of self-awareness and self-compassion. This can help individuals build resilience and coping skills that can be applied to other areas of their lives.

Using Art as a Tool for Self-Discovery and Emotional Healing

Art therapy can also be a powerful tool for individuals to engage in self-discovery and emotional healing. Through the creative process, individuals can explore their inner thoughts and feelings, and gain a deeper understanding of themselves and their pain experience. This can lead to a greater sense of self-acceptance and self-understanding, and promote emotional healing and growth.

Art therapy can also help individuals process difficult emotions and experiences related to their pain. By creating art, individuals can externalize their emotions and thoughts, and gain a new perspective on their pain experience. This can help individuals release pent-up emotions, and develop new ways of coping with their pain healthily and constructively.

In conclusion, art therapy and creative expression can be powerful tools for individuals living with chronic pain. By engaging in artistic activities, individuals can explore their emotions, reduce stress, and improve their overall well-being. Through the creative process, individuals can develop new coping strategies, gain insight into their pain experience, and promote emotional healing and self-discovery. Art therapy offers a unique and holistic approach to managing chronic pain and can be a valuable addition to a comprehensive pain management plan.

23

Chapter 23: Financial Wellness and Chronic Pain: Navigating Costs and Resources

Chronic pain can have a significant financial impact on individuals and families. From medical expenses to lost income and reduced productivity, the costs associated with managing chronic pain can quickly add up. Understanding the financial implications of chronic pain is crucial for effectively managing these costs and accessing the resources needed to support ongoing treatment and care.

Understanding the financial impact of chronic pain on individuals and families

Chronic pain can lead to a range of direct and indirect costs that can strain finances and impact overall well-being. Medical expenses, including doctor visits, medications, procedures, and therapies, can quickly become a significant financial burden for individuals living with chronic pain. In addition, the effects of chronic pain on daily functioning and quality of life can lead to reduced productivity at work, increased absenteeism, and even job loss, further exacerbating financial strain.

For individuals and families living with chronic pain, it is important to take stock of the full range of costs associated with managing the condition, including both direct medical expenses and indirect costs such as lost income and reduced productivity. By understanding the financial impact of chronic pain, individuals can better prepare for and manage these costs, seeking out resources and assistance to help alleviate financial strain.

Strategies for managing healthcare expenses and accessing financial assistance programs.

Managing healthcare expenses is a critical component of navigating the financial impact of chronic pain. Individuals living with chronic pain can take steps to reduce medical costs by exploring cost-effective treatment options, including generic medications, physical therapy, and alternative therapies. It is also important to work closely with healthcare providers to develop a comprehensive treatment plan that addresses both the physical and financial aspects of managing chronic pain.

In addition to managing healthcare expenses, individuals living with chronic pain may also benefit from exploring financial assistance programs and resources that can help offset the costs of treatment and care. Many organizations and foundations offer financial assistance programs for individuals living with chronic pain, providing support for medical expenses, medications, and other related costs. By researching and applying for these programs, individuals can access the resources needed to support ongoing treatment and care.

Building resilience and stability through financial planning and resourcefulness

Building resilience and stability in the face of chronic pain requires proactive financial planning and resourcefulness. Individuals living with chronic pain can take steps to protect their financial well-being by building emergency savings, creating a budget, and exploring cost-saving strategies for managing healthcare expenses. By developing a financial plan that accounts for the costs associated with chronic pain, individuals can better prepare for and navigate the financial challenges that may arise.

Resourcefulness is also key to managing the financial impact of chronic pain. Individuals living with chronic pain can explore creative solutions for reducing costs, such as negotiating with healthcare providers for lower fees, seeking out discounts on medications, and exploring alternative therapies that may be more cost-effective. By taking a proactive and resourceful approach to managing healthcare expenses, individuals can better navigate the financial challenges of living with chronic pain.

In conclusion, the financial impact of chronic pain on individuals and families can be significant, but by understanding these costs, developing strategies for managing healthcare expenses, and building resilience through financial planning and resourcefulness, individuals can better navigate the financial challenges of living with chronic pain. By taking a proactive and informed approach to managing finances, individuals living with chronic pain can access the resources and support needed to support ongoing treatment and care, ultimately improving their financial well-being and quality of life.

24

Chapter 24: Animal-Assisted Therapy for Chronic Pain Patients

Animal-assisted therapy (AAT) is a growing field that has shown promise in helping individuals manage chronic pain. The benefits of interacting with animals in this context are numerous, and research has demonstrated the positive effects of AAT on pain perception, emotional well-being, and overall quality of life for chronic pain patients.

The Benefits of Interacting with Animals in Managing Chronic Pain

The bond between humans and animals is a powerful one, and the presence of animals has been shown to reduce stress, anxiety, and depression in individuals with chronic pain. Interacting with animals can help to distract patients from their pain, provide comfort, and promote relaxation. This can lead to a decrease in pain perception and an improvement in mood, ultimately enhancing the patient's overall sense of well-being.

Studies have also shown that spending time with animals can increase levels of oxytocin, a hormone that promotes feelings of bonding and trust. This can help chronic pain patients feel more connected and supported, which can be especially beneficial for those who may be experiencing isolation or loneliness due to their condition.

Examples of Animal-Assisted Therapy Interventions and Their Effects on Pain Perception

Various types of AAT interventions have been used to help chronic pain patients manage their symptoms. One common approach is animal-assisted activities, where patients engage in activities such as petting, grooming, or playing with therapy animals. These interactions can help to improve mood, reduce stress, and provide a sense of companionship.

Another form of AAT is animal-assisted therapy, where trained therapy animals work with healthcare providers to assist in the treatment of chronic pain. For example, therapy dogs may be used to provide physical support during rehabilitation exercises, or to help patients practice relaxation techniques such as deep breathing or guided imagery.

Research has shown that AAT interventions can have a positive impact on pain perception in chronic pain patients. For example, a study published in the Journal of Pain Research found that spending time with therapy dogs resulted in a significant reduction in pain intensity and an improvement in pain-related disability among individuals with chronic low back pain.

Guidance for Incorporating Animals into a Pain Management Plan

For chronic pain patients interested in incorporating animals into their pain management plan, there are several considerations to keep in mind. First and foremost, it is important to consult with a healthcare provider or therapist to determine the most appropriate AAT intervention for your specific needs and goals.

If considering pet ownership as a form of AAT, it is essential to choose an animal that is well-suited to your lifestyle and abilities. For example, individuals with limited mobility may benefit from owning a small or low-energy pet, while those with allergies or sensitivities may need to carefully consider the type of animal they bring into their home.

For those interested in therapy animals, it is important to work with a reputable organization that follows best practices for animal-assisted therapy. Therapy animals should be well-trained, well-socialized, and certified by a recognized therapy animal organization.

In conclusion, animal-assisted therapy can be a valuable tool in the management of chronic pain. By incorporating animals into a pain management plan, whether through therapy animals or pet ownership, chronic pain patients can experience a range of benefits that may help to improve their quality of life and overall well-being.

25

Chapter 25: The Science of Pain: Understanding Neurological Mechanisms and Pathways

Pain is a complex sensory experience that serves as a crucial warning signal to protect the body from harm. The physiological processes involved in pain perception are intricate and involve a network of specialized nerve cells and pathways within the nervous system. Understanding the neurological factors contributing to chronic pain conditions is essential for developing effective pain management strategies. In this chapter, we will explore the science of pain, including the physiological processes involved in pain perception, the neurobiological factors contributing to chronic pain conditions, and insights from neuroscience research to inform holistic pain management strategies.

Overview of the Physiological Processes Involved in Pain Perception

Pain perception begins when specialized nerve cells called interceptors detect noxious stimuli, such as extreme temperatures, pressure, or chemicals, in the body. These nociceptors are located throughout the body and are activated in response to tissue damage or injury. Once activated, interceptors send electrical signals to the spinal cord and brain, where the sensation of pain is processed and interpreted.

The transmission of pain signals from interceptors to the brain involves a complex network of neurons and neurotransmitters. In the spinal cord, incoming pain signals are processed and modulated by various neural circuits before being transmitted to the brain. The brain then integrates these signals with other sensory information, emotions, and memories to create the subjective experience of pain.

Exploration of Neurological Factors Contributing to Chronic Pain Conditions

Chronic pain is a debilitating condition that affects millions of individuals worldwide. While acute pain serves a protective function, chronic pain often persists long after the initial injury has healed. The development of chronic pain is influenced by a variety of neurological factors, including changes in the nervous system and alterations in the processing of pain signals.

One of the key mechanisms underlying chronic pain is the phenomenon of central sensitization, in which the nervous system becomes hypersensitive to pain signals. Central sensitization can occur in response to persistent contraceptive input, such as in the case of injury or inflammation, leading to an amplification of pain signals and the development of chronic pain conditions.

In addition to central sensitization, other neurological factors can contribute to chronic pain, including alterations in the structure and function of the nervous system, changes in neurotransmitter levels, and dysfunction in pain-modulating pathways. Understanding these neurological factors is crucial for developing targeted interventions to effectively manage chronic pain.

Insights from Neuroscience Research to Inform Holistic Pain Management Strategies

Neuroscience research has provided valuable insights into the mechanisms underlying pain perception and chronic pain conditions, leading to the development of innovative pain management strategies. Holistic pain management approaches that target both the physical and emotional aspects of pain have shown promising results in improving pain outcomes and enhancing the quality of life for individuals with chronic pain.

One such approach is the use of mindfulness-based interventions, which have been shown to reduce pain intensity and improve pain-related disability by changing the way individuals perceive and respond to pain. Mindfulness practices, such as meditation and yoga, can help individuals develop greater awareness of their pain and learn to cope with it more deceptively.

Other holistic pain management strategies include cognitive-behavioral therapy, physical therapy, and integrative medicine approaches, such as acupuncture and massage therapy. These interventions aim to address the underlying neurological factors contributing to chronic pain and promote healing and recovery through a multidisciplinary approach.

In conclusion, the science of pain is a complex and multifaceted field that involves the interplay of physiological, neurological, and psychological factors. By understanding the physiological processes involved in pain perception, exploring the neuro-logical factors contributing to chronic pain conditions, and leveraging insights from neuroscience research, we can develop holistic pain management strategies that address the root causes of pain and improve outcomes for individuals living with chronic pain.

26

Chapter:26 References

List of Sources for Further Reading and Research

Turk, D. C., & Gatchel, R. J. (2019). Psychological approaches to pain management: A practitioner's handbook. Guilford Press.

Melzack, R., & Wall, P. D. (1965). Pain mechanisms: A new theory. Science, 150(3699), 971-979.

National Institute of Neurological Disorders and Stroke. (2019). Chronic pain: In depth. Retrieved from https://www.ninds.nih.gov/Disorders/Patient-Caregiver-Education/Fact-Sheets/Chronic-Pain-Fact-Sheet.

Institute of Medicine. (2011). Relieving pain in America: A blueprint for transforming prevention, care, education, and research. National Academies Press.

Jensen, M. P., & Turk, D. C. (2014). Contributions of psychology to the understanding and treatment of people with chronic pain:

Why it matters to ALL psychologists. American Psychologist, 69(2), 105-118.

Chou, R., & Shekelle, P. (2010). Will this patient develop persistent disabling low back pain? JAMA, 303(13), 1295-1302.

Gatchel, R. J., & Okifuji, A. (2006). Evidence-based scientific data documenting the treatment and cost-effectiveness of comprehensive pain programs for chronic non-malignant pain. Journal of Pain, 7(11), 779-793.

Shanthanna, H., Gilron, I., Rajarathinam, M., AlAmri, R., Kamath, S., Thabane, L., ... & Paul, J. (2017). Benefits and safety of gabapentinoids in chronic low back pain: A systematic review and meta-analysis of randomized controlled trials. PLoS Medicine, 14(8), e1002369.

National Center for Complementary and Integrative Health. (2019). Complementary, alternative, or integrative health: What's in a name? Retrieved from https://www.nccih.nih.gov/health/complementary-alternative-or-integrative-health-whats-in-a-name.

Jonas, W. B., O'Connor, B., & Deuster, P. (2015). The evidence base for integrative approaches in chronic pain. Explore, 11(5), 328-331.

Glossary

Chronic Pain: Persistent pain lasting longer than 3 months, often associated with a specific condition or injury.

Holistic Approach: A comprehensive approach to healthcare that considers the individual as a whole, including physical, mental, emotional, and spiritual aspects.

Psychosocial Factors: Psychological and social influences on pain perception and management, including beliefs, emotions, and social support.

Mind-Body Techniques: Therapeutic approaches that focus on the connection between the mind and body, such as meditation, yoga, and relaxation exercises.

Complementary and Alternative Medicine (CAM): Practices outside of conventional medicine that are used in conjunction with or as alternatives to traditional treatments.

Integrative Medicine: A holistic approach to healthcare that combines conventional and complementary therapies to address the physical, mental, emotional, and spiritual needs of the individual.

Neuroplasticity: The brain's ability to reorganize itself by forming new neural connections in response to learning and experience.

Biopsychosocial Model: An interdisciplinary approach to understanding health and illness that considers biological, psychological, and social factors.

Cognitive-behavioral therapy (CBT): A form of psychotherapy that helps individuals identify and change negative thought patterns and behaviors that contribute to pain and distress.

Multidisciplinary Pain Management: A comprehensive approach to pain management that involves a team of healthcare professionals working together to address the physical, psychological, and social aspects of chronic pain.

Self-Management Strategies: Techniques and skills that individuals can use to manage their pain and improve their quality of life, such as relaxation exercises, mindfulness, and goal setting.

27

Chapter:27 Conclusion

In this book, we have explored various strategies for holistic pain relief, recognizing the importance of addressing pain from a multifaceted approach. We have discussed the significance of incorporating physical, mental, emotional, and spiritual techniques to effectively manage pain and improve overall well-being. As we conclude our journey together, let us recap some key strategies for holistic pain relief and empower you to take control of your pain management journey.

Recap of Key Strategies for Holistic Pain Relief

Mind-Body Connection: It is essential to recognize the interconnections of the mind and body in managing pain. Mind-body practices such as meditation, deep breathing, visualization, and mindfulness can help reduce stress, enhance relaxation, and alleviate pain. By cultivating a positive mindset and practicing relaxation techniques, you can positively impact your pain experience.

Physical Therapy and Exercise: Physical therapy and regular exercise play a crucial role in maintaining mobility, strength, and flexibility, which are essential for managing pain. Engaging in gentle exercises like yoga, tai chi, swimming, or walking can improve circulation, alleviate tension, and enhance your overall physical well-being. Working with a physical therapist to develop a personalized exercise program can help you address specific pain-related challenges and improve your quality of life.

Nutrition and Supplements: A healthy diet rich in fruits, vegetables, whole grains, and lean proteins can support your body's natural healing processes and reduce inflammation, which is often associated with chronic pain. Incorporating anti-inflammatory foods, such as turmeric, ginger, garlic, and omega-3 fatty acids, can help alleviate pain and promote overall wellness. Additionally, consulting with a healthcare provider or nutritionist about incorporating supplements like magnesium, vitamin D, or glucosamine can provide additional support for managing pain.

Alternative Therapies: Explore alternative therapies such as acupuncture, chiropractic care, massage therapy, reiki, or aromatherapy, which can complement conventional treatments and offer additional pain relief. These holistic modalities work to balance the body's energy, release tension, improve circulation, and promote relaxation, leading to reduced pain and improved overall well-being. Be open to trying different therapies to find what works best for you and your specific pain management needs.

Encouragement for Readers to Take Control of Their Pain

Management Journey

As you navigate your pain management journey, remember that you are in control of your health and well-being. Empower yourself to advocate for your needs, communicate openly with healthcare providers, and explore various holistic approaches to find what works best for you. It is essential to be proactive in seeking out resources, support, and information that can help you effectively manage your pain and improve your quality of life.

Embrace a holistic approach to pain relief by integrating physical, mental, emotional, and spiritual practices into your daily routine. Cultivate self-care habits, prioritize relaxation, and stress management, and engage in activities that bring you joy and fulfillment. Surround yourself with a supportive network of friends, family, healthcare professionals, and holistic practitioners who can offer guidance, encouragement, and compassion as you navigate the challenges of living with pain.

Remember that healing is a journey, and it is okay to seek help, try new approaches, and adjust along the way. Be patient with yourself, practice self-compassion, and celebrate small victories as you progress toward holistic pain relief and improved well-being. By taking an active role in your pain management journey and embracing holistic strategies, you can empower yourself to live a fulfilling, vibrant, and pain-free life.

In conclusion, I encourage you to embrace holistic pain relief as a comprehensive and empowering approach to managing pain. By incorporating physical, mental, emotional, and spiritual techniques, you can cultivate a deeper understanding of your pain experience, enhance your overall well-being, and reclaim control over your health and quality of life. Remember that you are not alone in your journey, and there are resources, support, and solutions available to help you thrive. Embrace the power of holistic pain relief, and embark on a path toward healing, resilience, and vitality.

www.ingramcontent.com/pod-product-compliance
Lightning Source LLC
Chambersburg PA
CBHW070839260726
48660CB00005B/2091